Testimonials

Christine Stevens, Ub Drum - With years of experience at agape Idris Has created a powerful tool that combines spiritual practice and drumming I highly recommend it With years of experience teaching internationally Idris has created a program that combines drumming and spiritual practice for everyone. I recommend it.

Michael B Beckwith, Founder - Agape International Author Spiritual Liberation & Life Visioning. It is my honor to say that a great instrument of healing and inspiration is in our midst. His name is Idris Hester. Through this instrument was birthed Drummunication a pathway of revelation, enthusiasm, and wholeness. For those who are fortunate enough to partake, Life will never be the same. Let the joy times roll!

Rickie Byars Beckwith, Director of Music - With Idris Hester, it all begins with the One and on the One. In DRUMMUNICATION as in life, Idris is a messenger/guide who shares how and why Rhythm is fundamental to living a balanced and joyful life. A journey with the one who aligns in this way will be fascinating -for sure and healing -for real.

Dafi Shanti, Intuitive LMFT – Author of Brain Surgeons Don't Do Facelifts. For anyone ready and willing to open to this incredible transmission of light Idris will guide you through the journey of the soul and tap into or rather drum into your awareness the heart soul connection.

DRUMMUNICATION

A Transformational Experience

Revolution to Evolution

The Power of The Drum

A Miracle Man

IDRIS HESTER

ISBN: 1543056644
ISBN 13: 9781543056648

DEDICATION

I dedicate Drummunication: A Transformational Experience book to the Creator, Creative source, God of it all.

A very heartfelt deep appreciation to daughter Natasha JesSara Hester, for your unconditional Love, understanding, Joy and Pleasure that you bring to myself, family, friends, and planet. Thank you for the message that you brought to me when you came to this earthly plain, and in always helping me to remember who I am.

It is an honor, joy, pleasure, and privilege to dedicate this book to all the Master drummers, percussionist in this universal place, and higher spirit guides of rhythm, that have given, and sacrificed themselves, to using drums and percussion to promote perfect health, wellness, and healing. The material in this book is published as a tribute and in deep gratitude and thanksgiving to the steadfast commitment spirit, beauty, peace, love, and light that is within each of us as individuals, groups, and all drummers globally and beyond out of the darkness that we have been dealing with for such a long time.

A large portion of this information, knowledge, and wisdom has been shared with us through many Masters, especially as of recent.

I dedicate this book also in deep gratitude to some of his Drum & Percussion influences are, Olatuji Babatunde, Mongo Santamaria, Eddie (Bongo) Brown, Ralph McDonald, Larry Washington, Poncho Sanchez, Karl Perazzo, Raul Rekow, Alex Acuna, Tito Puente, the Escovedas, Buddy Rich, Joe Morello, Art Blakley, Billi Cobham, Stix Hooper, Harvey Mason, Ed Thigpen, Omar Hakim, Gerry Brown, James Allen, etc.

This dedication goes without so many words, to all the medical health institutions, doctors, nurses, health specialist, practitioners, health care students. Especially the Neurosurgeons and their teams which performed invasive surgeries on me.

Dr. Glenn Kindt: University of Michigan, Ann Arbor MI, Dr. Leslie Cahan: University of California, Los Angeles CA, Dr Lance Altenau: Sharp Scripps Medical centers, San Diego CA, Dr Keith L. Black, and Dr Gabriel Hunt: Cedar Sinai, Beverly Hills CA, PYSD Veronica Porche, Cedar Sinai for the many years of Psychotherapy, Hypnotherapy, Guidance counseling, Life Coaching.

I very special thank you to the Agape International Spiritual Center, Ministers, Practitioners, Congregants, and their family and friends

ACKNOWLEDGEMENTS

I Acknowledge the Creator, Creative source, God of it all with Gratitude and Thanksgiving. I am expressing my deep gratitude and thanksgiving to all my family, friends, and people around the world who have participated and supported the work that has been channeled through me.

I express my deepest gratitude and thanksgiving for members of the various drum organizations, Remo, Pearl, Toca, Latin Percussion, Meinl, Gon Bop, Tama, Ludwig, Gretsch, Sonor, Paiste, Zildjian, Pro Mark, Alesis, Vater, Drum Corp International, Percussive Arts Society, etc. Thank you for working so hard in making sure the drummers and percussionists have what is needed to express the healing power of the drum, to raise the human consciousness.

A very special deep heartfelt thank you to Dafi Shanti, LMFT, Intuitive Energetic therapist and healer in addition being the author of 'Brain Surgeons don't do Facelifts,' for her dedication in assisting and the preparation for expansion of *Drummunication: A Transformational Experience* throughout our planet. You have been instrumental in supporting the mission and miracles of Love which appear in all the Drummunication sessions globally.

All 12 Step Programs: AA, NA, CA, Alanon, Naranon, ACA, Every family and friend throughout this planet who support the recovery process. Special thanks, Hank W. and Lynn, Sherman H., Cornish H., Pam J., Zayid, and Pam T., Musa, and Sandy K., Mustafa, and Jennifer N., Malik and Darlene, Philip B., Daryl B. (RIP), Derrick H., Glenn D. All living in and out of the fellowships.

A special thank you with gratitude and thanksgiving to Rising Consciousness Center team members Psychologist Maya Shakti, Visionary Meditative Teacher Shiv, and Intuitive LMFT Dafi Shanti.

Thank you, all my family members, through all the years of supporting me through all my trials and tribulations, the good times, and the not so good times. So very Grateful and

Thankful to my parents, Sarah Hester, Lewis Hester, with deep sincerity and

appreciation for all that you have done for me and the siblings, Lawrence, Toni, Theron, Michael, Mark, Martin, Kevin, and Donald (RIP).

A special thank you to Talya for stepping up for me in a time of need, as well a thank you to Eillia for presenting smoothness.

Thank you, Sandra Zislis for the Amazing photography, and graphics.

Sandy Spiritual Nurse Sandy Manuel also for Graphics and social media post.

A very special thank you for my childhood, life long friends. Friends whom loved me unconditionally, supported me through many traumatic horrendous, self-defeating experiences, right or wrong, good, or bad, positive, or negative. Different or indifferent, tolerant, or intolerant. Hilyet Sample (Hitchie), Willie Morgan, Tommy Weathers, Curt Wilson, Craig White, Tony Smith, Bruce Harris, Jake Sampson, Grady Walker, Jim Jones, Hoover Sisson, Gregory Irwin (Waller), Willie Brown, Donald Jones, Kenyatta Weathers, Marilyn Wernet, Georgina LeHurray, Finese Williams, Garland Williams, Betty Delph, Jackie Holmes, Renee Chapman, Theresa Gladney, Patsy Sampson, Gregory Husband, Nate Williams, Terry Powell, Billy Norris, Johnny Love, Elgin Bennett, Charlie McCann, Dave Weatherwax, David Dudt, Ron Hively, Johnny Weatherwax, Gail Weatherwax, Ronnie McDonald, Daryl Parker, Tony Dungy, Maurice Mobley,

PREFACE

I, we, suggest that before you begin to read each chapter of the material in this book, take a moment to go into the sacred place within you that only you know of, which is a part of your uniqueness. Feel your pulse and heartbeat. Ask the power within you to increase your knowledge, wisdom, and understanding.

DRUMMUNICATION AFFIRMATION

Our pulse and heartbeat connect us.
We create the rhythm of life that radiantly flows
through the universe,
permeating absolute perfect health, wellness, and
healing for wholeness,
reawakening us to God, ourselves, and others spiritually,
mentally, physically, and emotionally.

Idris Hester

OUR PULSE AND HEARTBEAT CONNECT US

How are you doing? How are you feeling? How are you *being*? Are you energized? Are you relaxed? Ups, downs, highs, and lows? I would like to follow up with you, the participant, with a new program engineered and designed to change the way you think and feel about yourself and others. *Drummunication: A Transformational Experience* is a revolution to evolution. It is about perfect health, wellness, and healing for wholeness, as music therapy, using drums and percussion. Should you have any questions or comments, please feel free to contact me. Your presence is a heartfelt experience in wanting to change and be a better you. Thank you for all the support in purchasing this book. We look forward to seeing you in your local city to have a *Drummunication: A Transformational Experience* workshop. May we be graced by your participation. Please feel free to pass this on. Please be advised this process works, spiritually, mentally, physically, and emotionally. Peace, light, love.

HAVE GREAT EXPECTATIONS WITH YOUR JOURNEY

During your process and programming with *Drummunication: A Transformational Experience*, expect to develop a greater spiritual, mental, physical, and emotional higher understanding of the power of the drum and a new concept of your relationship with a universal mind power, the creative source of all good. *Expect almost immediately to have your life and affairs manifest this changed consciousness.* I wish to emphasize *you* must do it.

No one can do it for you.

And so, it is.

The Power of the Drum
Healing through Drums and Percussion
Individual and Group Empowerment Drumming
Sessions

TABLE OF CONTENTS

INTRODUCTION

Drummunication: A Transformational Experience

Shamanic, Angelic Sound Wellness and Healing Drumming Stages

This book is designed and engineered for you to achieve maximum health, wellness, and healing for wholeness, using drums and percussion as primary tools.

This is a personal, heartfelt call for you to remember the following:

<u>**Stage one,**</u> is a brief description of how *Drummunication: A Transformational Experience*, the book, came to be.

<u>**Stage two,**</u> we venture into something about me—stories and biography.

<u>**Stage three,**</u> we will move into the heart of the book. *Drummunication: A Transformational Experience* uses drums and percussion to promote your perfect health, wellness, and healing for wholeness.

<u>**Stage four,**</u> I added a way to help you expand yourself spiritually, mentally, physically, and emotionally. *Drummunication: A Transformational Experience*

Drumming Stage.

<u>**Stage five,**</u> gives you information on what it is to be a practitioner and on the six-step spiritual mind treatments, or affirmative prayer. This part of the book is most important to keep you knowing the correlation with spirit and the physical as one. The truth about the power of the drum uses the *Drummunication: A Transformational Experience* affirmation.

Our pulse and heartbeat connect us; we create the rhythm of life that radiantly flows through the universe, permeating absolute perfect health, wellness, and healing, for wholeness, reawakening us to God, ourselves, and others.

You will see the correlation between these stages of the book, how the stages are integrated and overlap one another, and why it was presented. This will help you see why *Drummunication: A Transformational Experience* came through this way.

Stage six, is about information on the sound aspect of drumming, with you experiencing your drumming either listening or playing along with the *Drummunication: A Transformational Experience* CD.

Stage seven, Closing

This book is not written traditionally, as other books are. This book is written for readers to have their own unique *Drummunication: A Transformational Experience*. Peace, light, love.

STAGE ONE

About Drummunication: A Transformational Experience

The Vision and Visioning

This vision is truly divinely inspired by a spiritual being in a human incarnation. This is a very special spirit who, in fact, has been divinely chosen to do radiant things. She came to me from the radiant light and through her constant spiritual relationship with God, inspiration, knowingness, intelligence, genius, love, caring, and kindness. The mother!

For a period now, it has been revealed to me to write about my experience, strength, and hope—through strong spirit, right thinking, and a higher conscious contact with the perfect power within (God)—as to where I am now. I am in the image and likeness of God, here to be of maximum service to God, myself, and especially others.

Drummunication: A Transformational Experience came through.

I am beginning to remember how to understand who, what, and why I am, and so will you.

I have been graced with seven neurosurgeries—four invasive brain tumors removed and two invasive surgeries to clear staph infections, with one cerebral embolization—and the spiritual, mental, and physical aspect of what these things were all about is coming through the gateway, opening wider, and the portal is deeper. I am receiving the final messages.

These messages came from other writings (books): *Going into the Light, Being in the Light, Coming from the Light, Living with the Light, Going through the Tunnel,*

Experiencing Freedom from Self, *It Comes to This*, *I'm Still Here*, and *What You Don't Know about Me*. I have a much deeper meaning now. This writing must be shared with those who are interested in recovering from not remembering who they really are. Out of this, *Drummunication* revealed itself through my experiences.

Remembering

I can remember myself being a great master humanitarian, engineer, designer, philosopher, mystic, shaman, healer, physician, father, drummer, percussionist, musician, and so much more. I remember running free, being free to be who I am.

I also remember seeing the spirits and souls of others. I remember being abused, forced to say things I did not think or feel. I remember being told I was mischievous, bad, evil, not of this world, curious, crazy, inventive, highly creative, troubled, and mental and that I was not going to be anything.

I can remember at later times in my life coming across different people from my past life and seeing some of the persons that had said negative things to me. For the life of me, I just could not understand what they were speaking of, because for me, I was surely none of these things. I would pretend that I was invisible or that I didn't exist. However, I'm grateful for the words that were being said by others. I have become the opposite of the negative words through drumming prayers and drums, meditative drumming, and intentional drumming. The negatives became positives through using *Drummunication: A Transformational Experience.*

I remember that despite all the things going on around me, it was just natural for me to forgive—and in some cases, forget—some of the things that happened.

I remember this deep, warm feeling inside me that was present all the time. I could only love everything and all, instantly, right now, with no thoughts or feelings of judging. I would say to myself I will love unconditionally. I would cry on the inside a lot, being mindful and careful about whom I would share these feelings with. Most of the time, I would not share these inside tears with anyone; I would internalize these feelings. I am forever a forgiving being.

A Message

Greetings, radiant spirit light drummers. Know that if you have a pulse and a heartbeat, I believe that you are a drum. You have the frame, which is your bone structure; you have the skin, your flesh; and your pulse and heartbeat provide the rhythm.

Are you ready to experience the power of the drum through drumming?

Drummunication: A Transformational Experience wants to happen through you.

This message is coming to you from spirit guides, angels, and the one presence for your loving support. This is to happen for your perfect health, wellness, and healing for wholeness, with anyone or anything that you meet at a sacred gathering place. Some people are ascended, in ascension, transcended, making a transition, and ready and available to get started, teach, and learn.

Drummunication: A Transformational Experience supports perfect health, wellness, and healing for wholeness spiritually, mentally, physically, and emotionally, teaching facilitation by me, a "miracle man," Idris Hester. This drumming integrates shamanic and angelic sound wellness and healing using drums and percussion. The shamanic deals with all the sounds of nature, past, present, and future. The angelic comes from ethereal and auric fields of energy. I discovered an integration with shamanism and angelics. Drumming uplifts and energizes one spiritually, mentally, physically, and emotionally. You will also experience a process called guided drummeditation healing, which is a very important part of the process of *Drummunication: A Transformational Experience.* The deeping is clearing and cleansing energy. It is about expanding all the goodness of your qualities, spiritually, mentally, physically, and emotionally, into the remembering and knowing of one's whole self. You will become more aware and conscious of your gifts and talents; the deeping comes as a result of this awareness and consciousness-raising process. The power of the drum. Revolution to evolution.

STAGE TWO

A venture into something about me

About the Author

Please review and embrace this information with the love of a mother. I believe that you will see my experience as a major strength that would bring to this planet a way to successfully use the many principles in the text that is *Drummunication: A Transformational Experience*. In these writings, you will find strong communication, organization, and ways to help us all live in this world united and to really see the power of one, based on using the principles in this book.

I am Idris Hester, founder of *Drummunication: A Transformational Experience*, a *Drummunication* facilitator, HealthRHYTHMS group empowerment drumming session facilitator, chief consciousness officer, light barrier, urban shaman, and angelics worker. It is very special to teach wellness and healing through drums and percussion—a revolution to evolution, the healing power of the drum—with my peers. Know that all things work for the good for all.

Yes! I am a witness to the powers of prayer and meditation in correlation with the wellness and healing power of drums and percussion using the *Drummunication:*

A Transformational Experience principle to process spiritual, mental, physical, and emotional maladies, negativity, guilt, shame, blame, anger, and so on. The process is about your well-being and other people who are in your life circles. This is a scientifically based program with spirit being my guide through many ways and things. The program was created to reeducate or educate others and to pass on these important shifts in our consciousness through my experiences and education. I have also lectured and spoken on these experiences to various groups. Hopefully I will be able to continue to share some of my background, education, and experience with wellness and healing through drums and percussion (and computers also).

I welcome the opportunity to be selected for your team and look forward to hearing from you. Thank you for your time and consideration.

By education and training, I am a world-class master percussionist/drummer, professor of music and spiritual sciences, music director/therapist, drummunicator, HealthRHYTHMS group empowerment drumming session facilitator, spiritual healer, urban shaman, angelic guidance servicer, alcohol/chemical substance-abuse counselor, and electrical/civil engineer and designer. With these accomplishments, the title I am most passionate about and dedicated to is that of *Shamanic Angelic wellness facilitator* (SAWF). I was born and grew up in Jackson, Michigan, small town seventy miles west of the Motor City—Detroit, Michigan, home of the internationally famous Hitsville USA, Motown Records.

At a very young age, I begin displaying technical skills; human-association skills; leadership; highly creative art skills in painting, drawing, and working with clay and ceramics; and a very high interest in music, especially drumming. I was very athletic and did seasonal sports, cross-country running, football, wrestling, fencing, baseball, and track and field, as well as many other things.

The art of music was the most fascinating, especially drumming. I started performing and entertaining as a drummer and percussionist at the early age of eight, starting in elementary school and then in junior high school, high school, and college. These experiences saw me performing with marching bands, concert bands, orchestras, jazz bands, and churches. Then I changed to performing various styles of music in bands: rock and roll, rhythm and blues, blues, funk, jazz, Latin, and fusion crossovers. This experience has had a great effect on the writing of this book. I have performed all styles of music and entertained people with many professional local and traveling groups throughout the country. I have had many musical accomplishments throughout my career. One major accomplishment for me and for individuals and society as a whole is teaching a wide diversity of people from many cultures, nationalities, communities, and families *Drummunication: A Transformational Experience*—revolution to evolution, the power of the drum, and healing through percussion—instructing people to be able to care for themselves and to become one with each other, keeping in mind that the healing has a community base. The outcome for the students has been overwhelmingly positive.

I have been influenced by the teachings of these great drummers and percussionists: Mongo Santamaria, Eddie (Bongo) Brown, Ralph McDonald, Larry Washington,

Poncho Sanchez, the master Dr. Henry Gipson, Earl DeRouen, Karl Perazzo, Raul Rekow, Alex Acuna, Tito Puente, the Escovedas, Buddy Rich, Joe Morello, Art Blakey, Billy Cobham, Stix Hooper, Harvey Mason, Ed Thigpen, Omar Hakim, Gerry Brown, Ricky Lawson, Jerry Rodgers, and others. I also have a love for composers/ arrangers such as Quincy Jones, Yanni, Henry Mancini, Mozart, Tchaikovsky, Bach, Beethoven, Burt Bacharach, Duke Ellington, John Coltrane, W. S. C. Handy, and Undine Smith Moore. All the jazz greats have had a positive influence on my performing style.

I am known as one of the premier universal, complete percussionists, with a definite worldly style and sound of my own, with a natural burst of energy and a flair, with the smoothness of silk and the coldness of ice, spiritually, mentally, physically, and emotionally.

My home base is Los Angeles, California.

Shamanic Angelic wellness facilitator is a title that I feel does not represent fully what services I provide; however, it serves its purpose for now. My history and life experiences have amply qualified me for this position to work with other mental health clients and staff. I am the survivor of seven invasive neurosurgeries, operations, the removal of four brain tumors, and three surgeries associated with the invasive brain-tumor operations. I have found many pre- and post-self-healing techniques using *Drummunication: A Transformational Experience*, the guided drummeditation healing method, the science of mind six-step spiritual mind treatment, new thought, ancient wisdom, and spiritual principles; there is literally no one on the planet who has survived such experiences. I was pronounced dead on many separate occasions and garnered great wisdom during my time spent on the other side of the veil. I have profound and vivid memories of being in this unconditionally loving divine light, and I call on this light to help guide me and individuals I work with. Because of my powerful connection with spirit, I can channel significant amounts of information for people, revealing to them their gifts and talents. I am truly a beacon of light who continuously, patiently, and lovingly guides people through projects, relationships with partners, clients, and the world to go forward in their growth and development.

Ever since my first neurosurgery thirty years ago, because of my health situation I was told by doctors that I would most likely not survive surgery, and if I did, I stood a very strong chance of being in a vegetative state, handicapped or disabled, having many mental disorders and issues for the remainder of my life. However, I have learned or am learning how to live with these options. I courageously underwent each surgery and worked my way back to a fully functional life, relearning how to walk and talk all over again each time. I was diagnosed with my fourth brain tumor on March 6, 2007. I decided not to undergo another surgery and have successfully healed this condition with the application of my own healing programs and the assistance of some world-renowned healers. In fact, it is because of my own miraculous healing experiences with drums and percussion that I have developed this amazing program, *Drummunication: A Transformational Experience*, to help move others into perfect health, wellness, and healing for wholeness, no matter what their present spiritual, mental, physical, and emotional conditions are.

It is my dream to one day live in a world where the title *Shamanic Angelic wellness facilitator* is as common as "president" or "CEO." I know that as individuals and companies with similarities step into higher consciousness, this planet can truly be a place where peace and love abound, and all people are being the greatest manifestation of their beings!

I see this as my opportunity to continue providing my present skills and experience for better mental health, substance abuse, emotional and behavioral disorders, wellness, and health; to be a voice of help for people who have problems with PTSD, OCD, alcohol, drugs, addictions, gambling, anger, and eating disorders; to provide wellness and health for all individuals, helping them identify behaviors and problems related to their specific needs; and to hold sessions for individuals, families, and groups of people.

I have always been active in underserved areas, whether race, creed, color, ethnicity, religion or lack of religion, discrimination, or prejudice has been used against people in these areas. Because of my activities in the Los Angeles area, I have received citations of commendation for my service and work. I received one for all the service and time I provided for chemical dependency and alcohol abuse in the inner city. I received another for working in the Pacific and Asian American community. I also received an award from the All Peoples Organization for being involved in change for everyone. I received another award from the Amity Foundation for helping former inmates, parolees, reach their highest potential to reach their goals and become productive members of society, using my position as a counselor and my counseling and music therapy experience. Over 90 percent of clients were prescribed various medications for psychological issues. Most are dual diagnosed. I am an inspirational/motivational speaker, life coach, and voice for all mentally challenged persons like me. The clients I have assisted include but are not limited to substance abusers, chemical- and alcohol-dependent people, institutionalized parolees, juvenile delinquents, people with PTSD, OCD, ADD, or ADHD, and Neighborhood Watch programs. I have a high interest in health consumers and thus have been a critical participant in groups that have a direct interest, involvement, or investment in health, something that is valuable to the employees and customers of business concerns with mental-health policy processes. I will be able to provide a strong speaking voice for mental-health clients, so we can be heard on all issues concerning clients and public policies affecting them in the government, the media, and the community.

I have engineered, designed, created, and developed plans of action for the Asian American Drug Abuse Program

(AADAP), the Young Mens Chistian Association (YMCA) youth program through Communnity Employment Training Act (CETA), and the Amity Foundation. I have directed, managed, coordinated, and facilitated program staff who acted as consultant advisors in this process.

Wellness and Health
Drummunication is a strong advocate for wellness and health. I do assessments; individual, group, and family wellness and healing sessions; crisis wellness and health; grief counseling; substance-abuse assessment and counseling; suicide assessment and prevention; and critical-incident stress debriefing.

Leadership
Drummunication can assist with management, supervision, and problem solving. *Drummunication* teaches and helps you coordinate projects including developing the project action plan, timeline, and budget.

Valuable, Treasured Experiences

My past experiences were put here in this book to help the reader get a better understanding of wellness and healing through drums and percussion.

I came from a hopeless state of mind, body, and soul, proving that something can come from nothing.

Having seven major neurosurgeries for invasive brain-tumor removal has been difficult. Using drummunication along with the HealthRHYTHMS protocol, I have truly experienced the therapeutic value of wellness and healing through drums and percussion. It reduced stress, reduced worry, heightened my senses, and allowed me to become more articulate, especially in my motor skills. The guided imagery gives me a relaxed state of wellness.

Using drums and percussion as a wellness and healing tool has relieved me from the negative effects of alcoholism and drug addiction. The individual, social, and economic relief was given back to me by experiencing and teaching wellness and healing through drums and percussion, doing drum circles, caring, and sharing, which brought about a sense of community and service within the community.

Also, I have had the luxury of being relieved from incarceration in the penal system. My drums and percussion instruments were allowed into the penal system. I was able to teach and learn more through this experience, being a part of the process of wellness and healing through drums and percussion.

I am labeled "a miracle man," urban shaman, HealthRHYTHMS facilitator, and shamanic angelic facilitator who does individual and group empowerment drumming sessions. My experiences and services include public speaking, lectures, workshops, and seminars for groups and individuals.

I have collaborated with many different types of organizations as to the usefulness of *Drummunication* for mental-health clients and how to be in alignment with them.

I educate, lecture, teach, and train for perfect health, wellness, and healing for wholeness using drums and percussion. One modality used is the HealthRHYTHMS group empowerment drumming session program protocol (REMO Drums Corporation).

I am a professional HealthRHYTHMS facilitator, drummunicator, shaman, inspirational speaker, percussionist, and spirit guide. I was educated by Dr. Barry Bittman, who is a neurologist, author, international speaker, award-winning producer, director, and inventor. Dr. Bittman is CEO and medical director of Mind-Body Wellness Center. He holds degrees in social work and music therapy. Dr. Bittman pioneered a new paradigm for treating the whole person. He is one of the principal investigators of the human genome. A genome is an organism's complete set of DNA, including all its genes. Each genome contains all the information needed to build and maintain that organism. In humans, a copy of the entire genome—more than three billion DNA base pairs—is contained in all cells that have a nucleus.

I was also educated by Christine Stevens, MT-BC, MSW, MA, a board-certified music therapist. She holds a master's degree in social work and music therapy.

I have experience working at various institutions, educating, lecturing, teaching, and training for perfect health, wellness, and healing for wholeness using drums and percussion, *Drummunication: A Transformational Experience*, and the HealthRHYTHMS group empowerment drumming session program protocol (REMO Drums Corporation). I demonstrate how group drumming has certainly survived the test of time, while the scientific community is just beginning to develop a rudimentary understanding of the biological, psychological, and sociological benefits of this multifaceted recreational music-making activity. I have made several television appearances, including on CBS, NBC, and PBS. Additionally, I am an alcohol/substance abuse counselor. I created a universal drummunication transformational experience system. I am an electrical/civil designer, professional percussionist, practitioner, and ministerial student in training (AGAPE International Spiritual Center).

Diversity is one of the major assets of this process; it involves all races, creeds, colors, genders, religions, and nonreligion.

Growing up

I grew up in Jackson, Michigan, a sacred place and on sacred land with awesome, amazing individuals. It was during a time when everyone treated each other like family. School was mandatory!

Growing up in Michigan, I always felt a power, a strong presence, so strong I could not feel it but could see it. I can remember clearly there was a mysticism, mastery, beauty, magnificence, and joy about it. It was so indescribable and immeasurable, with such an unconditional love. I tended to pay more attention to it than to my surroundings. Today I know I was closer than close with God and living a high knowing of my spirit.

For me there was a broken home, in which I was verbally, emotionally, and physically abused. Living this life took me on many of these journeys. All is forgiven and well. I know today that the total sum of my life experiences has me kept me here today before you amazing people, to share some of my gifts and talents with you.

I could feel the rhythm pulsing through my existence and every fiber of my body. It was an indescribable charge and surge of energy, yet it felt to me permanent, everlasting, forever eternal. My body was shaking, vibrating uncontrollably. I could feel and hear the pulse and heartbeat of myself, others, and the universe. Yes! I was afraid, but only for what seemed like a brief moment that appeared in time. Questions came up through me: What was that? Where did it come from? And why me at this time? From that moment on, I was constantly moving, shaking my hands as though drumming, even though I had no idea what drumming was. All the time I was beating on things, anything that had a sound to it or that a sound would come from. Whom was I to talk with about this experience? For deep inside, I knew that no one would get it. I did try it once or twice. It is the power of the drum.

A Revealing Matrix Idris

Through my feelings came a heavy sadness, a reawakening and awareness of the Native American, Egyptian, African, Trinidadian, Russian, and Irish beings in myself. I am highly in touch with the technologies of the ancients and ancestors that are living through me and with the power of the drum, rhythm, and sound.

Our pulse and heartbeat connect us.

I am clearer on my purpose and intentions for being here. I am processing information so fast that I have to practice remembrance.

I must use the technologies to express this knowing that our pulse and heartbeat connect us, the power of the drum, revolution to evolution.

Dimensions

From the many travels and journeys, physical, non-physical, in body, and out of body, I have experienced and had many events of the human experience as one being, whole and complete with the one, I have come to understand and strongly believe that I came into a powerful vision, a great, mystical, magical idea that I see and that feels real.

We are taught about multiple dimensions and different levels. However, what was revealed to me is that there is only one dimension (accumulative), which has everything in it. The only dimensions that exist are what man has created. This increases a sense of separation, more labeling and putting things in boxes.

STAGE THREE

Heart of the book

A historical view

For centuries people have used drumming to release stress, raise their spirits, enhance clarity, and focus, and develop a culture of cooperation and community. It is a powerful team-building method. *Drummunication: A Transformational Experience* is designed to energize and engage individuals and to unify community spirit through group empowerment drumming sessions.

Feeding the Hungry Soul

As we move into the twenty-first century, it has become apparent that our society relies largely on technology and materialism to sustain us. Yet through all our technological advances, there persists a deep and ever-present need to find happiness and fulfillment, meaning, and purpose in ways that technology simply does not offer. Despite its impressive marvels, technology does not have the capacity to provide us with meaning or purpose. As we have embraced technology, we have forgotten that one of the great needs we have as individuals is to be heard, to find and create simplicity, and to make connections of the heart, mind, and soul with others. The drum fulfills all these needs.

The drum provides us with an ancient form of communication, one that does not rely on the articulation of words but that uses a much more basic language: our emotions expressed through sound. When you hit the drum hard, it can be an expression of anger. When you hit the drum softly, it can be an expression of fear or contemplation. It's this basic simplicity of expression that makes the drum a perfect means for children and others who may censor or repress their emotions because they fear judgment or feel unsure of how to express their feelings in words.

The drum seems to awaken the recognition of a spirit within. Yet often the soul's calling goes unnoticed. We feed our bodies when they get hungry, yet we do not see the signs and cues that our souls give us when they're hungry. The emptiness and the hopelessness within our society serve as signs and symptoms that our collective soul needs to be fed.

Our soul is not fed by reading negative newspaper stories and viewing news accounts of pain and suffering on television. Our soul is not fed by technology, no matter how extraordinary the advances may be. Our soul is not fed by closing our minds and hearts to love and its many rhythms and manifestations.

The soul is fed through turning our attention within, through connecting with others in ways that reflect depth and purpose, and through play and laughter. The soul is nurtured through connections of the heart. The drum provides all these needs. The hand drum serves as a touchstone to our deepest nature. It is both a symbol of our spirit and a vehicle to transport us into it.

And so, it is.

Hand Drums and Healing

When the word "drum" is uttered, most people imagine a person sitting behind a drum set, crashing out rhythms while a band plays on. Until recently, the words "drum" and "transformation" were rarely used in the same sentence. Yet the humble, relatively unknown hand drum—not the drum set of smoky bar fame—is fast becoming an instrument used by people of every age for personal transformation, psychological and physiological healing, and creating community.

The use of the hand drum in relationship to healing is certainly not new. The hand drum has been used for thousands of years in celebration, rituals, and ceremonies. However, the merging of science with the healing qualities of the hand drum is a relatively new development. Per anecdotal reports and current research, the hand drum and its rhythms have been instrumental in improving illnesses when medical science had few answers.

Hand drums are drums from around the globe that are played not with sticks but, as common sense would suggest, with one's hands. These drums, which represent a plethora of countries and continents, include the African djembe, the South American Surdo and Pandeiro, the Middle Eastern Doumbek, the Japanese Taiko drum, and the Irish Bodhran and Frame drum, along with many others.

Drum and Percussion Wellness and Healing Workshops

Drummunication: A Transformational Experience provides many individual and group lessons on specializing in living rhythms for promoting spiritual, mental, physical, and emotional balance for living life.

All people are usually welcome to these workshops.

Research

While group drumming has certainly survived the test of time, the scientific community is just beginning to develop a rudimentary understanding of the biological, psychological, and sociological benefits of this multifaceted recreational music-making activity. A landmark controlled scientific investigation by Barry Bittman, MD, and colleagues in *Alternative Therapies in Health and Medicine* (January 2001) demonstrated statistically significant positive cell-mediated immune system changes that correlated with one-hour group drumming sessions using the HealthRHYTHMS group empowerment drumming protocol. This unique approach has been successfully used as a well-accepted, cost-effective strategy in a host of clinical outcome-based programs for individuals facing the challenges of heart disease, cancer, chronic lung disease, and asthma. New research using the HealthRHYTHMS group empowerment drumming protocol enhanced with the Yamaha Clavinova demonstrated statistically significant reductions in burnouts and improvements in mood states for long-term care workers (Bittman et al., *Advances in Mind-Body Medicine*, Fall/Winter 2003). Projected cost savings (by an independent healthcare economic impact firm) to the long-term care industry were actually exceeded by real-world findings.

Learning Objectives

Drummunication: A Transformational Experience gives a hands-on training program that has been carefully designed to offer you an unforgettable, interactive, life-changing opportunity for discovering and sharing the incredible rhythms that are yours alone. During our enjoyable, intensive interdisciplinary workshop, we will explore key evidence-based elements, potential benefits, and widespread applications for incorporating this multifaceted approach in your work. As we practice the basic structured elements of this protocol, our learning-by-doing approach will progressively reveal countless operational insights and clinical pearls critical to the future success of your program, supported by a comprehensive, easy-to-follow training handout with manuals. Musical experience is not required. You will quickly learn how to successfully introduce, integrate, and transform through *Drummunication: A Transformational Experience* group empowerment drumming sessions in a variety of health and wellness settings.

Philosophy

Group drumming is not about inspiring successful drumming—it's about inspiring successful living. Group drumming is not about exceptional performance—it's about exceptional support and personal expression. Group drumming is not about teaching people to play—it's about giving people permission to play. Group drumming's best facilitators are not only talented musicians—they are caring, compassionate, and intuitive guides. Group drumming is not about acquiring technique—it's about sharing for the sake of personal *empowerment.*

Who Should Learn about This Process

Regardless of prior musical experience, if you're searching for meaning and purpose in your life through creative musical expression, the innovative *Drummunication: A Transformational Experience* process is for you. While past participants have included doctors, nurses, music therapists, psychologists, social workers, members of the clergy, practitioners, activities directors, drug and alcohol counselors, and family therapists, we welcome non–health professionals who are willing to work collaboratively as team players with health-care professionals. If you're in the health and wellness fields and wish to help people move beyond their perceived boundaries, this program is likely to be just what the doctor ordered!

Effects of Group Drumming

Here are some reasons that drumming can be used in prevention and for interventions for anxiety and depression, social resilience, and inflammatory immune response among users of mental-health services.

Health Reasons to Start Drumming

1. **It makes you happy.** Drumming releases endorphins, encephalin, and alpha waves in the brain, which are associated with general feelings of well-being and euphoria.

2. **It induces deep relaxation.** In one study, blood samples from participants who participated in an hour-long drumming session revealed a reversal in stress hormones.

3. **It helps control chronic pain.** Drumming can serve as a distraction from pain. And it promotes the production of endorphins and endogenous opiates, the body's own painkillers.

4. **It boosts your immune system.** Studies show that drumming circles boost the immune system. Barry Bittman, MD, has shown that group drumming increases natural T cells, which help the body combat cancer as well as viruses, including HIV/AIDS.

5. **It creates a sense of connectedness.** Drumming circles provide an opportunity for synchronicity to connect with other like-minded people.

6. **It aligns your body and mind with the natural world.** The Greek origin of the word "rhythm" is "to flow." Drumming allows you to flow with the rhythms of life by simply feeling the beat.

7. **It provides a way to access a higher power.** Shamans often use drumming as a means to integrate mind, body, and spirit.

8. **It releases negative feelings.** The act of drumming can serve as a form of self-expression. When held, negative emotions can form energy blockages.

9. **It puts you in the present moment.** While drumming, you are moving your awareness toward the flow of life. You cannot be caught up in your past or worried about your future.

10. **It allows for personal transformation.** Drumming stimulates creative expression. Drum circles provide a means of exploring your inner self and expanding your consciousness while being part of a community.

STAGE FOUR

Drumming Stage
A way to help you expand yourself spiritually,
mentally, physically, and emotionally

Drummunication Definition

Drummunication: Using rhythmic and sound vibrations to express feelings or emotions into a thought from the heart; speaking, visioning, or communicating without words. One of the highest forms of nonverbal communication. These questions are to be answered by you, the reader.

1. What are *your thoughts* about this definition?

2. What are *your feelings* about this definition?

How to Use This Information

It is beneficial to practice drumming regularly and develop a sense of connection that the drum can impart between the inner you, your spiritual potential, and the outer world.

The drum is a doorway through which you can connect and through which you can be connected with spirit.

This is a journey that will never end and will continue to surprise you, so take time to drum. When we drum, we drum from the center of our beings, and so we will learn together the meanings through which drums came about and how drumming can affect your relationships with everything. Then we can learn to drum. Close your eyes and imagine that you are with us; place yourself as a part of the drum circle.

This is an excellent opportunity to bring the rituals of drumming back into your life. If you persist with your practice, the rewards will be beyond words, and your life will be forever richer and more beautiful because of it.

You will also learn how to use the drum to keep your living space clear and how to create a meditative atmosphere in your home. You will learn how to use drumming to shift major issues such as fear, resentment, and anger. You will learn how using your drum can help you pass through and accept the natural biological and spiritual changes that take place in our lives, the rites of passage. The joy of a new life at birth, the gentle release of a loved one at the end—the drum will enrich these beautiful transitions.

Through the power of drums and percussion, you will notice the wonderful instrument of healing your drum is and how it can be used in a variety of ways.

Study and practice repeatedly with intention.
Try this. Beat the drum and wait for guidance; actively seek guidance through the slow, gentle connection that the drumbeat gives you. It does not take long; it is the intention that counts. Strike the drum, move into the desire to serve clearly, and let your mind begin to speak to the spirit. Ask the spirit to give you words so that a message can be conveyed.

Take me away from ignorance, and let me be guided.

Notes:

Introduction to Healing through Drums and Percussion

The longest journey begins with the first step.

—Ancient proverb

In this case, the journey starts with the discovery of the spirituality of drumming. Drumming connects you with your bones, your heartbeat, and your natural rhythms. You connect with the drum by holding it close to your heart and letting your feelings transfer into the drum. When we breathe, we all beat on a common drum. The drum acts as a mediator between the drummer and the spirits, between space and time, between power and people. The drum can change the direction of life, calling everyone's attention and eliminating distractions.

When we drum, our consciousness, focus, and clarity are out, and our intuition is acute. We feel for the atmosphere of love, we feel for the spirit, and we wait and call for the spiritual space to be filled with the *wakan* (all that is holy and spiritual). The drum acts as a channel, a method of centering and projecting the attention into areas of consciousness that are inaccessible in normal life.

For me, through my many life experiences, drumming has been an opportunity to serve spirit, the very source of all our lives and all that surrounds us on this beautiful planet.

I need to feel inspiration; I need to feel as if I am coming from the real me, where love rests, and there is no fear.

People from all cultures have drums. They make drums from wood, trees, and skin. Black, yellow, red, and white—we all have drums, and we don't remember who made them first. Every day is holy and spiritual, not just one day of the week. When you drum, you connect with the spirit. The drum contains everything and all; all the natural and spiritual world is in the drum.

Study and practice repeatedly with intention.
Try this. Beat the drum and wait for guidance; actively seek guidance through the slow, gentle connection that the drumbeat gives you. It does not take long; it is the intention that counts. Strike the drum, move into the desire to serve clearly, and let your mind begin to speak to the spirit. Ask the spirit to give you words so that a message can be conveyed.

Take me away from ignorance, and let me be guided.

Notes:

Spirituality and the Drums

*The world where there is nothing but the
Spirit of all things, this is the real world that
is behind this one, and everything that we see
here is somehow a shadow from that world.*

—*John G. Neihardt*

The beat of the drum has a quickening effect, which is so basic in its relationship to the human organism that it unifies and brings together the consciousness of all who are in listening range. No matter what we are doing or thinking, when we begin to hear drums beating, we hear the same sounds, and it affects us usually in the same way: we must pay attention.

Drumming connects with our whole beings, existence, and natural rhythms. The beats bring us down to earth, out of our heads, into our feelings. Rhythm pushes through emotions and intellect and lifts the spirit.

Drumming can be used to do the following:

- To center us as individuals with one another, to connect in the spirit as one as we affect one another's lives
- To remove negativity in our spaces and give us clean spiritual energy
- To allow us to pray, giving thanks and praise for all we need

- To direct us straight to the source for our meditations
- To help us to have a better understanding of the state of trances we go into and out of, knowing that it is OK
- To just take away negative emotions
- To break us free from being stuck with our spiritual energy and purpose; to raise our consciousness of our environment and how it can affect us
- To bring about a oneness spiritually in a group and to bring us together with a sense of direction

When we feel the spirituality of the drum, we must start by looking deep within ourselves. It is from here that the spirit comes. It is behind our eyes.

Study and practice repeatedly with intention.
Try this. Beat the drum and wait for guidance; actively seek guidance through the slow, gentle connection that the drumbeat gives you. It does not take long; it is the intention that counts. Strike the drum, move into the desire to serve clearly, and let your mind begin to speak to the spirit. Ask the spirit to give you words so that a message can be conveyed.

Take me away from ignorance, and let me be guided.

Notes:

History of the Drum

From North America to Siberia, Australia to Africa, China to Britain, wherever you travel on this majestic globe, the drum is or has been used in spiritual celebrations. From prehistory to the modern industrial era, the beat of the drum has measured time. In greeting the dawn or welcoming the birth of a child, in praying for rain or celebrating at a marriage celebration, in drumming to the setting sun or gently bidding farewell to a passing friend, the drum has measured the passage of time, holding us firmly in the present, reminding us of our hearts and connection through rhythm and beat to something that we must stay connected to.

In the book *The Secret Power of Music*, David Tame describes ancient Chinese orchestras. What mattered was to use earthly tones as an aid in reaching spiritually inward and upward to the source of all tone and all creation.

Shamans of all cultures have used and still use the drum as their means of traveling through different layers of reality.

Storytelling with the Drum

Before the complexity of modern music, wandering societies would draw together around the fire, using the drum for dance, song, and storytelling. The drum circle stood for love, unity, and healing. The drum was used to unite people: drumming, like a pulse, reinforced their group identity through sound.

Study and practice repeatedly with intention.
Try this. Beat the drum and wait for guidance; actively seek guidance through the slow, gentle connection that the drumbeat gives you. It does not take long; it is the intention that counts. Strike the drum, move into the desire to serve clearly, and let your mind begin to speak to the spirit. Ask the spirit to give you words so that a message can be conveyed.

Take me away from ignorance, and let me be guided.

Notes:

The Power of the Drum in Today's Times

*Your children are not your children; they
are the sons and daughters of life, longing
for itself. You may give them your love, but
not your thoughts. You may house their
bodies, but not their souls. For their souls
live in the house of tomorrow. For life goes
not backwards nor tarries with yesterday.
You are the bows from which your children
as living arrows are sent forth.*

—*Kahlil Gibran, The Prophet*

The timing cycles govern our lives: sixty seconds, minutes, hours, days, weeks, months, and years. The timing cycles that were set for us govern our lives. We arise in the morning and go to sleep at night, consistently exploring the timing events. Too late or too early, what suits us and what does not suit us, timing cycles are related to our comfort and happiness. Eating, recreation, exercise, and many other activities occur at regular intervals. With drumming, there is no continuous melody; it is the breaking up of silent space with sound at regular intervals. It is this regular form that comforts and soothes us, the new people.

The first sound that we heard was our mothers' heartbeats as we floated in the amniotic sac months before our births. For most of us, this must have been the ultimate comfort zone, and we want, deep down, to retain that level of stability. Our lives are going through many fast-paced changes, so any way that we can bring back that experience, the feeling of being secure, feels good for us. The more that this can be experienced in our group drumming, the more cohesive the feeling of security. Drumming brings the individual to feel like a part of the group.

Nowadays, we easily lose touch with our feelings and natural rhythms by being involved with mental and intellectual activity. As an example, children spend more time in school in front of a computer screen or at home in front of the television and less time feeling and aligning themselves to the natural rhythms of nature and the family. It is our responsibility to shift the boundaries and push the conditional limitations of society.

Study and practice repeatedly with intention.
Try this. Beat the drum and wait for guidance; actively seek guidance through the slow, gentle connection that the drumbeat gives you. It does not take long; it is the intention that counts. Strike the drum, move into the desire to serve clearly, and let your mind begin to speak to the spirit. Ask the spirit to give you words so that a message can be conveyed.

Take me away from ignorance, and let me be guided.

Notes:

About the Drum

The drum, for the most part, is handheld and is made of either hollowed-out wood or steam-bent wood or a metal tube that is molded into a hoop. Rawhide leather is stretched over the frame and secured on all sides. When the skin is dry, it tightens. When it is dry, the drum sound is high, hollow, and hard. When the skin gets damp, the skin loosens, and the sound becomes low, dull, and soft. You can get many sounds from the drum depending on the environment.

When you are in a drumming group with lots of drums working together or crossing over in sound, your drum will find a life of its own. A group is a wonderful place to learn, where you can start to understand that the drum evolves into an extension of yourself and your inner self as you gain confidence in your drumming. When people are drumming together, a connection with unity and relationships will develop with others, as long as the ego is out of the way. Drumming is also fun; it allows everyone a chance to learn and excel. Using the drum for healing brings about a different spiritual experience, where your level of skill as a drummer becomes directly connected with your personal growth. The more you drum, the more you relax your mind, body, spirit, and physical self, and your spirit becomes open. Your drum becomes a part of the journey you are taking, helping you shift through physical, emotional, and spiritual limitations using sound, vibration, and movement.

Drumming is a wonderful exercise. As you beat away on your drum, let your body relax and become part of the movement. It is good to try to let yourself sing, chant, and even dance.

The power of intent transports your drumming experience out of the comfort zone. Be patient and strong as you drum, drawing on the inner power to direct you.

Study and practice repeatedly with intention.
Try this. Beat the drum and wait for guidance; actively seek guidance through the slow, gentle connection that the drumbeat gives you. It does not take long; it is the intention that counts. Strike the drum, move into the desire to serve clearly, and let your mind begin to speak to the spirit. Ask the spirit to give you words so that a message can be conveyed.

Take me away from ignorance, and let me be guided.

Notes:

Cleansing, Blessing, Dedicating, and Caring for the Drum and Practicing the Self-Healing Powers of Drumming

Now that you have your drum, you will need to awaken the energetic relationship between the two of you. This already started in the process of the drum coming to you in a sacred manner. That sacredness needs to be built on, not only through regular use but also through cleansing. Keep your drum in a dry place and in a sacred area.

When you awaken your drum, you give it life, connecting yourself and the drum in a sacred relationship. So you may want to choose a special time alone or with a friend. Prepare yourself beforehand through prayer and meditation, remembering why you wanted a drum and what you desire to do with it. Do you want to use it for healing, or is it going to be used primarily for celebration? Decide what you and your drum are going to do together; let this purpose come to you over a few days prior to your opening ceremony.

As you now drum, draw in your dedications and intentions, invite blessings into your drum, let yourself go into the experience, and focus on calling into the drum all the goodness, holiness, and power that you can experience. When the experience is over, give a vocal prayer of gratitude to all spirits present. Your drum is now awakened and ready to be used for healing. This sets the standard for the future use of the drum.

Study and practice repeatedly with intention.

Try this. Beat the drum and wait for guidance; actively seek guidance through the slow, gentle connection that the drumbeat gives you. It does not take long; it is the intention that counts. Strike the drum, move into the desire to serve clearly, and let your mind begin to speak to the spirit. Ask the spirit to give you words so that a message can be conveyed.

Take me away from ignorance, and let me be guided.

Notes:

Learning the Drum

When you receive your drum, consider it a gift. You now have some information on how to care for your drum. You should have something in your thoughts as to where the drum comes from, what the drumbeats are about, and where the beats are to be sent. Relax and get in touch with your breath and your prayer. It may be easier if you close your eyes. Start by gently beating on your drum.

Finding Your Own Personal Beat

Everyone has a beat or drum rhythm that he or she naturally falls into. This is what you want to explore first. The beat that has come to you will be a strong foundation that a lot of your future drumming will come from. Keep things slow, and then work into stronger drumming. Let yourself look into sound, and look for simplicity; be cautious of complexities with drumming.

Sounding Your Drum

Every drum has a different sound. Explore your personal beat, and move around, hitting your drum in different areas. Find where you get the best sound for yourself. Rub your drumskin heads; use your fingernails; tap the outside of the drum; hit the rim. Use bass tones, slap tones, and medium tones.

Drumming in Nature

Go into the woods, go to the beach, and explore the different sounds. Watch how the drum changes with different trees and the ocean sounds. Find your personal beat, and observe how it varies with the differences. Sometimes you may feel nothing. When this happens, move around; your drum may really open you up. Let yourself give your drumming as a gift, and let your spirit connect with the spirits of the place. *Awesome* experience.

Drumming with Others

Meet with other drummers, and explore each of your personal beats. Listen as you drum, and follow. Observe how each person is able to experience and express himself or herself more fully through drumming. Let your sound come through when you feel guided. This is an opportunity to find your connection to spirit. Explore drumming and keeping beat with your less dominant side; you will be beating strength into your spirit within the support group.

Study and practice repeatedly with intention.

Try this. Beat the drum and wait for guidance; actively seek guidance through the slow, gentle connection that the drumbeat gives you. It does not take long; it is the intention that counts. Strike the drum, move into the desire to serve clearly, and let your mind begin to speak to the spirit. Ask the spirit to give you words so that a message can be conveyed.

Take me away from ignorance, and let me be guided.

Notes:

Clearing and Cleansing the Way by Drumming

"Hanta yo" means "clear the way." Remove all that is blocking your way to the spirit, inspirations, and creativity; have a clear route of expression. Drumming will help you to accomplish this. Drumming clears away all dross and conditioned responses so that something from deep inside can come out. The beat of the drum is like a sweeping broom: the vibrating sounds not only enter the ears to be heard, which clears all the thoughts of the mind, but also pierce the congestions of the aura, moving the air around the body, bringing in clarity, and dispersing confusion of the mind.

Our limitations are a high percentage and commonly due to the fear of change. Pain! This means that we pay more attention to what is in our limited thinking, more so than to what we want to create.

Pain makes you move from your comfort zone and seek solutions, and it is always your choice where you would like to go with a remedy. You may see pain as not your responsibility and wish to be a patient and present your problem to a doctor, whom you have been conditioned to look on as a superior person. By accepting others' advice and medicines that you are expected to take, you often give away your own power and autonomy.

Let us perceive this another way. Let us now give away our power. Let us see the pain as a way in which we can move from fear to love. Pain says, "Look at me!" Eventually you will find that you won't be able to run from it forever. Pain makes you change many ways and things; pain makes you change your posture and your habits. It makes you look at the things you have buried deep inside yourself mentally, spiritually, and physically, emotions or beliefs you have wanted to keep a secret. You just want to know what this pain means; you want to know what changes will help bring you closer to being a happier person. You will find that the pain you feel is not so much a negative as a positive and necessary part of being alive and open to change.

This information is meant to help you change your attitude toward dealing with pain.

Study and practice repeatedly with intention.
Try this. Beat the drum and wait for guidance; actively seek guidance through the slow, gentle connection that the drumbeat gives you. It does not take long; it is the intention that counts. Strike the drum, move into the desire to serve clearly, and let your mind begin to speak to the spirit. Ask the spirit to give you words so that a message can be conveyed.

Take me away from ignorance, and let me be guided.

Notes:

Intentional Drumming with Prayers

The energy, focus, and, above all, the heightened consciousness of the people present in the drum circle are drawn together and can be directed toward healing, prayer, and gratitude. This is often a more powerful way to pray and direct the feelings and prayers you want to project out to different people. This collective consciousness is anchored by the drum and links the heart pulse of the holy earth to the hearts of individuals, leaving no room for manipulation and hysteria.

It is most important that the prayer be directly linked to spirit and that it be selfless. We must learn to serve this power that fills us with each breath of life. When we pray as individuals or in the collective, we are creating radiant light.

First, understand clearly why you are praying. When you are ready, start the drumming. Create a special place; make it clean.

Feel comfortable with silence, and then start to pray aloud when you feel the power is coming through you.

As you pray, call in the collective energy of the drum circle so you are all focused on the same outcome.

If others want to make a prayer, invite them to do so. You do not have to pray for too long. Spirit prefers swift, direct prayer, so feel for the time to stop.

When you are ready to stop, emphasize the qualities of trust and gratitude, because it is the collective faith and hope that calls spirit to answer our prayers.

Study and practice repeatedly with intention.
Try this. Beat the drum and wait for guidance; actively seek guidance through the slow, gentle connection that the drumbeat gives you. It does not take long; it is the intention that counts. Strike the drum, move into the desire to serve clearly, and let your mind begin to speak to the spirit. Ask the spirit to give you words so that a message can be conveyed.

Take me away from ignorance, and let me be guided.

Notes:

Drumming Meditation

*Every so often the Heart Says, "Fill me" and
this can cause great anguish if you don't
know how. To me, the priority must be to
listen, to listen to what the heart has to say.
To listen to what this voice has to say to me.*

—Maharaji, Reflections

Meditation is the process of going inside ourselves and contacting the source. The source is the same for us all. It is a continuous flow of life that starts somewhere deep inside us all. It comes up in a loving way through our senses. With the drum, we can go infinitely into a place where there is such stillness that you feel you have seen or experienced it forever. Listen to what the heart must say.

Start a meditation process by finding somewhere quiet, where you will not be disturbed.

Bring your drum close to you. Gently begin to beat your drum. Find your beat and listen. Embellish; enjoy all the sounds coming through your drum. Feel the contact between the body of the drum and your own body. Allow yourself to feel at one with the sounds being produced. Relax and always continue to take deep breaths. Let the resonance of the drum and your breath come together.

As you begin to experience the uniting of the drumbeat with your own internal rhythms, let the drumming slow down as you look for your heartbeat.

Let go of your focus on the drum; stay looking and listening inside. What do you see? What do you hear? What do you feel? Allow yourself to go deeper into the beat. Do not worry if the drumming stops; stay focused on the inner experience. If you become distracted, and you need to get back to meditating, just focus on the drumbeat again. When the time comes for you to stop meditating, bring yourself back to drumming a steady rhythm.

A Drumming Meditation

In group meditations, the drum is a wonderful vehicle for holding space and keeping the participants in focus. This is a relaxing and therefore gentle process to be handled with sensitivity and clear intent.

Study and practice repeatedly with intention.
Try this. Beat the drum and wait for guidance; actively seek guidance through the slow, gentle connection that the drumbeat gives you. It does not take long; it is the intention that counts. Strike the drum, move into the desire to serve clearly, and let your mind begin to speak to the spirit. Ask the spirit to give you words so that a message can be conveyed.

Take me away from ignorance, and let me be guided.

Notes:

Drumming Away Fear, Anger, and Sadness

*I think we are moving in a circle, or maybe
a spiral, going a little higher every time,
but still returning to the same point. We
are moving closer to nature.*

—*John Fire Lame Deer*

The drum is a powerful tool for letting go of feelings of anger, fear, and sadness. Part of the process of learning to walk with me through *Drummunication: A Transformational Experience* and healing through drums and percussion is to experience difficulties. Life is like the sea: the tide comes in when you take your first breath, and the tide goes out when you take your last breath. The sun rises, and we all warm up and run around; then the sun goes down, and we must cuddle up and stay warm. All life is circles within circles, and we are very much a part of the circle.

Fear is the emotion that many human disorders are based on. The way to heal all fear of diseases is to send out love to the cause of the fear. With your drum, focus your attention on the source of your fear or on whatever you can establish as the closest thing to its essence. Drum into the place, and pour into it all the spiritual, mental, and physical energies you can find. If you still feel fearful when you are finished, take a break, and then start the process again.

Anger is an emotion where feelings need to be expressed but have been repressed. You will need to let out the frustration that cannot find an exit. Again, it is a matter of timing. Let the drum bring you back into time with the whole. Hold the drum, and send your prayer into your source as you beat, and with powerful intent, ask to be released from your false expectations. Ask through the drum how to let the anger disperse.

Sadness is a sickness; it is long and lingering and forces us to hold onto the past. Sadness is white and cold and needs the warmth of the rising sun in the east to see there is new growth, opportunity, and experience coming as the constant wave of the present keeps moving forward. Breathe with the drum, and find a drumbeat as close to the breath as possible. Push the sound through the breath into the source, and ask to have the pain taken away. Sing a song as you drum; in the song, ask to have the pain taken away.

Study and practice repeatedly with intention.
Try this. Beat the drum and wait for guidance; actively seek guidance through the slow, gentle connection that the drumbeat gives you. It does not take long; it is the intention that counts. Strike the drum, move into the desire to serve clearly, and let your mind begin to speak to the spirit. Ask the spirit to give you words so that a message can be conveyed.

Take me away from ignorance, and let me be guided.

Notes:

Introduction to Mindful Drumming

Through mindful drumming, we can get in touch with our deeper selves and thereby feel connected with the humanity of other people as well. The benefits of mindful drumming include many components. Here are a few: empowerment, the cultivation of deep listening, a chance to tap the higher power within, community building, inner peace, deep happiness, and heightened self-esteem.

I don't believe in accidents, because you are here. My hope is that this class will guide you to a deeper unfolding and knowing of your amazing spirit, which you cover up. The purpose of this class is to help you unleash the power that lies within you as you connect with the community around.

Mindful drumming will provide a natural, effective, and fun process for liberating us and removing the blocks to our wholeness. Through our direct experience of the twin realities of rhythm and vibration, we can be transported into states of happiness, peace, joy, faith, love, gratitude, compassion, and so on.

You will learn through the teachings and your own experiences how to unleash the strength of your spirit and come into your full power as a human being as you learn to be mindful of rhythm, vibration, and sound. You will learn the simple methods of mindful-drumming meditation, which is as easy as learning to pay attention to the rhythm of your own footsteps.

Study and practice repeatedly with intention.

Try this. Beat the drum and wait for guidance; actively seek guidance through the slow, gentle connection that the drumbeat gives you. It does not take long; it is the intention that counts. Strike the drum, move into the desire to serve clearly, and let your mind begin to speak to the spirit. Ask the spirit to give you words so that a message can be conveyed.

Take me away from ignorance, and let me be guided.

Notes:

Mindful Drumming: Unleashing the Human Spirit Practice to Unleash the Human Spirit: Experience the Basics of Mindful Drumming

1. Turn off all electronic devices and any distracting sources. Get out your drum, or if you do not have access to a drum, imagine your thighs to be a drum, or use a tabletop. Sit quietly in a comfortable position.
2. Gently tap out three even counts on your drum, or whatever you are using as a drum, with the palms of your hands. One, two, three, and on the fourth beat, clap your hands.
3. Repeat this simple rhythm of three taps followed by a hand clap. Always maintain equal measurements between counts. Please use a slow or moderate speed. Continue this pattern at least ten times.
4. Next, you can experiment with keeping this simple rhythm going for a minimum of three minutes, or longer when you have time, and the time is *now*.

Study and practice repeatedly with intention.
Try this. Beat the drum and wait for guidance; actively seek guidance through the slow, gentle connection that the drumbeat gives you. It does not take long; it is the intention that counts. Strike the drum, move into the desire to serve clearly, and let your mind begin to speak to the spirit. Ask the spirit to give you words so that a message can be conveyed.

Take me away from ignorance, and let me be guided.

Notes:

Guided Drummeditation Healing

Guided drummeditation healing is about expanding all the goodness of your qualities, spiritually, mentally, physically, and emotionally. It helps you help yourself *energetically* to clear all old ideas, thoughts, and paradigms of who you may have created yourself to be or think of yourself as being, as to how you must be to be peace, spirit, beauty, blessed, gratitude, compassion, joy, faith, love, freedom, and bliss. You will have an experiential experience using *Drummunication: A Transformational Experience*. We will be involved in music therapy and music as medicine and the healing power of the drum. Part of your experience will be to use musical instruments, drums, and percussion for beginners or masters in drumming. All are welcome to this forever life-changing experience with world-renowned master drummer/percussionist, urban shaman, spirit/intuitive guide, and chief consciousness officer Idris "the Miracle Man" Hester. What are your thoughts? Peace, light, love.

Study and practice repeatedly with intention.
Try this. Beat the drum and wait for guidance; actively seek guidance through the slow, gentle connection that the drumbeat gives you. It does not take long; it is the intention that counts. Strike the drum, move into the desire to serve clearly, and let your mind begin to speak to the spirit. Ask the spirit to give you words so that a message can be conveyed.

Take me away from ignorance, and let me be guided.

Notes:

A Time to Start

This is a time for reflection. It is a time to look back at the past weeks to see where you have come from to where you are in the present. With willingness, you can practice what you have learned in and out of class and bring this to a new place that is specially designed for you.

Use all the tools, and you will be there. Use the new support group you have. Thank you all for your relentless achievements and accomplishments. You are all awesome. You are now conscious of drummunication healing through drums and percussion and the healing powers of the drum, which you have initiated. Give yourself plenty of love, care, and kindness. You without a doubt are radiating these qualities as we wind down.

Take time daily to read something from this book; call someone in the circle with whom you have affirmed the unity of oneness.

Study and practice repeatedly with intention.
Try this. Beat the drum and wait for guidance; actively seek guidance through the slow, gentle connection that the drumbeat gives you. It does not take long; it is the intention that counts. Strike the drum, move into the desire to serve clearly, and let your mind begin to speak to the spirit. Ask the spirit to give you words so that a message can be conveyed.

Take me away from ignorance, and let me be guided.

Notes:

STAGE FIVE

Spiritual Growth Stage

Defining and Clarifying the Definition of a Professional Practitioner

This stage is included in *Drummunication: A Transformational Experience* to assist you in your spiritual practices and to give you a way to expand your drummunication process in recognizing all the attributes of God, to know that you know God. To unify that there is only one thing happening here, God. To realize that it is done, to be in the overflow. To be in an attitude of gratitude and thanksgiving, being grateful for what you have. To release, knowing the universal laws are activated constantly, working for the greater good of yourself and others. For you to know that God is all there is. You are being the expression of this power. This is the truth for all and everything, right now, as you write or say these words, affirming, confirming the one power, the one presence, as yourself and as the reader of this statement.

And so it is.

Who Am I as a Practitioner?

I am one of the greatest expressions of God, who is manifesting this almighty power through me as me. I am helping to raise the God consciousness of myself and others. I am practicing allowing God to express himself in all areas of life. And so it is, and so it shall be, and so it is done!

When I See Myself as a Professional Practitioner, What Do I See?

I see that the total sum of my life's experience is engineered, designed, and put into action by me, only to keep me on the path to what I am seeking. I see myself being of maximum service to God, myself, and others. I see nothing but the image and likeness of God manifesting itself through me. I am getting to practice these spiritual principles in a sacred and reverent way. I see myself always being in the spirit, being a mirror image for all to see who they really are. I see myself holding a high station and vibration coming from all my predecessors, professional practitioners who laid a path for me to follow. And so it is; so it is done. Amen!

What Is Seeking to Emerge in and through Me as I Begin This Journey?

One thing I know for sure is that I will get more practice in becoming a professional practitioner. My higher self, greatness, transcended mastery, mysticism, spiritual practices, evolving consciousness, and strong foundation are emerging through me through you. This is always and forever now!

I am so grateful at this time that excitement, love, joy, peace, happiness, abundance, prosperity, excellence, beauty, wonderment, creativity, wellness, healing, perfect health, and so many attributes of God are emerging right now! Grateful, meaning feeling or showing an appreciation of kindness; thankful.

Six-Step Spiritual Mind Treatment Using Drums and Percussion

In *Drummunication: A Transformational Experience*, we will approach this process using the six-step spiritual mind treatment, which is based on the Reverend Michael Bernard Beckwith's addition to the five-step spiritual mind treatment from the science of mind teachings.

During the process of a spiritual mind treatment, also known as affirmative prayer, scientific prayer, or simply "treatment," we come to the realization that within the universe there is one infinite, universal presence that permeates everything, and therefore this presence, being everywhere, must be right within us as well. With this attitude of mind, we reach an acceptance of new possibilities in life, and we are able to see, feel, and speak of the good we desire as already ours. Then we let the universe work its magic.

1. Give thanks for the perfect power (drumming from a place of thanksgiving).
2. Recognize the perfect power. Use your drum to affirm and confirm the one power. You are to strike the drum with authority.
3. Unify with the perfect power. Beat the drum with even spaces between the beats, holding the intention of one.
4. Realize the perfect power (choosing your good). Beat the drum with zest, zeal, vitality, and vigor.

5. Have gratitude for the perfect power (accepting your good). Go into the meditative drumming, being still on the inside.

6. Release the perfect power. Beat the drum from the place of knowing peace, spirit, beauty, gratitude, compassion, joy, faith, love, freedom, and bliss, being aware that this is all happening simultaneously, even though you may choose one or many of these affirmative words.

Have Great Expectations

Expect to develop a greater spiritual understanding and a new concept of your relationship with the universal mind power using drums and percussion, the creative source of all good. Expect almost immediately to have your life and affairs manifest this changed consciousness. I wish to emphasize that *you* must do it.

No one can do it for you.

And so it is.

Step 1: Give Thanks for the Perfect Power

The first step is accepting your good. This requires faith. Jesus said, "What things so ever ye desire, when ye pray believe that ye receive them and ye shall have them." This is where most people fail. They do not feel they are worthy of accepting the good that really belongs to them. All that the Father has is thine. You are indeed a son of God, beloved of the Father, and it is the Father's good pleasure to give you a healthy body, a happy life, and an abundance of all good things.

You need only accept them as coming from the one source, and they are yours. That which you accept or experience in mind will become manifest in your outer experience. If your heart's desire is born in love and does not harm anyone else, then you should be able to accept it confidently.

And so it is.

Notes:

Step 2: Recognize the Perfect Power

This is the second and most important step. It cannot be overdone. It means to recognize the power and presence of God right where you are and everywhere present within every part of life. Infinite good is everywhere present. Since infinite good is everywhere present, how can evil exist? Infinite love is everywhere present, like a loving parent, desiring your highest good, loving you with an everlasting love that encompasses everything that concerns you.

Divine love is power in your life, omnipotent power, all power, a power so great you cannot even conceive of it, a power for which nothing is impossible. All power includes wisdom and intelligence. Infinite intelligence knows the answer to your every problem and can bring order and right action into your life in ways you know not of. We recognize that the power is the source of all good and can provide us with the substance out of which it can be executed. It is wholeness, divine well-being, which manifests as physical and mental health and abundant supply.

If you are using the spiritual mind treatment to treat someone, realize that God is one infinite mind and that you are not separated from the person for whom you are using the spiritual mind treatment. Furthermore, you are not trying to change the other person; you are changing your thinking about that person. The perfect power within you and within all life knows how to bring perfect, right action into this experience.

The key *thought* in this first step is to recognize that God is everywhere present. You cannot become separated from God (good) for a single instant. You have only thought yourself separated. As we realize the omnipresence of God, we realize that there is no place where God—infinite good, divine love, perfect peace—is not. We do not have to make God happen. God already exists in fullness in every part of life. God is all-wise, all-knowing, and all-powerful and knows how to do all things for us in the right and perfect way.

And so it is.

Notes:

Step 3: Unify with the Perfect Power

Now we know of the existence of the perfect power, which is God. We have recognized the perfect power as being within ourselves and within all life.

Without us, God would not be expressed, for man is the image and likeness of God. This means that as persons of God, we have right within us the power, the intelligence, and the love of God. It is right where we are, and we are one with it. All things are possible for God through us.

To feel consciously unified with God, first surrender all the hate, anxiety, resentment, and negative thinking, and let the oneness of God's perfect life fill the mind. Forgive yourself and your brothers and sisters for every mistake. As long as we separate ourselves from another living soul, we separate ourselves from God.

Think to yourself: I am one with all life. I love my fellows and all life. I am one with the creative power of life. I am one with God's healing light. I am one with God's divine abundance. I am not separated from any part of life. I and the Father are one. God is living his perfect life through me now. All that God is I am in expression.

And so it is.

Notes:

Step 4: Realize the Perfect Power

Choose your good. Now, aware of the presence and power of God, we take the fourth step, which is to place into the mind the desire of the heart. Be relaxed in your choosing. *It is God's good pleasure to give you the kingdom.* The will of God for you is for an abundant, healthful, joyful, and happy life, because the will of God must conform to the nature of God, and the nature of God is love, joy, and life. Suffering, lack, torment, and sorrow stem from our own ignorance and lack of understanding of God.

In making your choice for yourself or for another, turn completely away from the old condition, the ill health, or the lack of abundance, and give your attention to the new choice. In other words, *start with the answer*, rather than the problem. Think about the desired perfection. Know that this perfection exists now in the mind of God.

Just as we plant a seed in the soil, we place the desire in the mind, knowing that the divine intelligence knows what to do to make it grow and bear fruit. It is important that we make a choice and stick to it. When we plant a carrot seed, we will not get a cantaloupe. We must know what we want and then let it come into manifestation. God knows how to bring it into our experience at the right and perfect time.

And so it is.

Notes:

Step 5: Have Gratitude for the Perfect Power

We speak, bring forth, from within ourselves a feeling of gratitude. Of course, the source of "all that is" does not need our gratitude to function; it is rather that an attitude of gratitude opens our consciousness to receiving even more good. As the law of the universe is such that what we focus on is what we manifest in our experience, when we are focused on the good that we already have, we can only attract more good—feeling or showing an appreciation of kindness and being thankful.

"I'm very grateful, thankful, and appreciative to you for all your help."

Receive or experience with gratitude. It is welcomed.

And so it is.

Notes:

Step 6: Release the Perfect Power

The sixth step is giving thanks for your good. Jesus gave thanks before the visible manifestation of the healing. As he stood before the tomb of Lazarus, he said, "Father, I thank thee that thou hast heard me," even before he commanded Lazarus to come forth. He not only accepted the healing but also was so sure that he gave thanks beforehand. The sixth step is really part of the fifth step, for it is an act of faith that strengthens your acceptance to the point where you really believe that it is done and can really release the entire situation to the Father within, who doeth the works. The sixth step is often called the releasing. As you give thanks, let go and let God.

And so it is.

Notes:

Review of Six Step Spiritual Mind Treatment

These are the six steps in a spiritual mind treatment. They constitute scientific prayer. The same thought sequence appears in the Lord's Prayer. When properly used and understood, the six steps accomplish a complete changing of the mind or consciousness.

We live in a spiritual universe, and every time we treat ourselves or another person, something is bound to happen. The idea is to persist until the mind has really changed and can accept the new idea. As we persist, there will be a fulfillment of our hearts' desires.

And so, it is.

STAGE SIX

Drumming Exercises Stage - Sound aspect of drumming

How to Use the *Drummunication* CD

You have just purchased the divinely inspired *Drummunication: A Transformational Experience* CD. The inspiration for this drumming CD comes through Idris Hester and Babies of the Universe.

Thank you for purchasing this CD. I want to personally affirm and congratulate you on showing up, paying attention, being truthful, and releasing all preconceived ideas about what you are about to experience with yourself and others in listening to and practicing with these amazing drumming recordings. My hope is that you will become more conscious of your loving, trusting, believing, and having-faith nature, as well as everything around you, and will listen to your spirit guides on the amazing journey you are about to experience.

Put in the CD, get comfortable, and become as still and quiet as you can. Breathe deeply; inhale and exhale. Allow yourself to move into your natural breathing pattern. Now listen to spirit, remembering there is no right or wrong way to do this. Should you be listening to the drumming CD, use the affirmative words that are the titles of each track as a reference point to set an *intention* for yourself and anyone who comes into your thoughts, as there may be many variations or relationships of the word you are using. Take, for example, the word "peace": listen to peace, listen for peace, think of peace, feel the peace, know peace, be peace, you are peace.

Now listen to the rhythm being played by the drum, feel the drum, and play your drum. You may play along with the drum. Improvise a rhythm to reflect your intention. Always remember there is no wrong way to drum. In the beginning of this process, you may feel as though you are not in rhythm. No worries; it is OK. Practice listening and drumming until you feel the peace of your inner drummer become activated. Drum for three to five minutes. Repeat this exercise as many times as necessary to achieve the maximum benefit.

Stop the CD. Close your eyes. Now breathe deeply, inhale the breath of God (receiving), and exhale the God breath (giving back). Listen to your inner self. Pay close attention to the space in between each breath. Ask spirit, what is the purpose of this peace? What is being called forth for me and others?

You will open up to the remembrance, "Our pulse and heartbeat connect us. We create the rhythm of life that radiantly flows through the universe, eternally permeating absolute perfect health, wellness, and healing for wholeness, reawakening us to God, ourselves, and others."

You are peace, spirit, beauty, blessed, gratitude, compassion, joy, love, faith, freedom, bliss, and so much more.

Drummunication: A Transformational Experience CD Drumming Title List

Introduction

1. Peace	03:56
2. Spirit	03:13
3. Beauty	03:29
4. Blessed	02:46
5. Gratitude	03:14
6. Compassion	03:09
7. Joy	03:16
8. Faith	02:59
9. Love	03:01
10. Freedom	02:47
11. Bliss	04:09

Closing

© *Drummunication: A Transformational Experience*
Website: www.drummunication.com
E-mail: idris@drummunication.com
Phone: (213) 663-4226
ASCAP. All rights reserved

STAGE SEVEN

Closing

Drummunication lesson

Dear Drummunicator, thank you so very much for taking the *Drummunication: A Transformational Experience Shamanic Angelic Sound Wellness and Healing journey. How exciting It is to now be of action for God, yourself and others optimizing using your gifts and talents. What a great time it is now for your process to evolve, ever expanding.*

Here is the final Drummunication lesson to practice. Because you have read this text book, the process below will assist in your wellness and healing. This is a no matter what, something that I suggest this lesson as necessary to be and do.

This lesson is to help give you a way to set intentions for yourself. To vision and to do visioning. To create in your mind's eye who you want to be.

Instructions

Thank you for simply being you. Here are the instructions to assist in your Spiritual growth. Here is a process to raise your conscious and heighten awareness.

Please write before going to bed 10 things that you are Grateful for No Matter What. Observe your behavior in doing so.

Inhale and exhale three times
Inhale the *breath of God* (receiving)
Exhale the *God breath (giving)*
Inhale the *breath of God* (receiving)
Exhale the *God breath (giving)*
Inhale the *breath of God* (receiving)
Self-tense up your muscles, hands, arms, legs, toes, neck, and shoulders, etc.
When doing the breathing exercise, it is important to pay attention to what is happening in between the inhale and exhale.
Exhale the *God breath (giving)*

Do 3 – 5 minutes of prayer and meditation (P & M)
Read the questions, study, contemplate, and do some reflection on your past, present, and future. Answer these questions one at a time and in order. Also, remember that this is not a I.Q., scholastic, comprehension, level, or aptitude test. The questions are infinite, and eternal. What comes through you will constantly change and expand

thus giving you more clarity about who you are, what you came to be and do.

Review what you have written. Without changing what you have written, get as still and quiet as you can, see what has come through you. As you observe your thoughts and what you are feeling. You are to celebrate for yourself after answer each question.

1. Who Am I?
2. What do I want?
3. Why do I want it? (Most important)

I offer to you to contact me after you answer each question through email. idris@drummunication.com

Remember that this Is about using your enlightenment. PLL

Idris

ABOUT THE AUTHOR

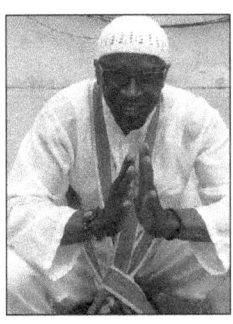

The founder of Drummunication: A Transformational Experience (DATE), author Idris Hester grew up deeply aware of the sacred rhythms of the universe, a pulse and heartbeat that seemed to pulse through him and with him.

Hester is a civil/electrical and electrical-design engineer. He is also a shamanic angelic practitioner and facilitator, master drummer, percussionist, health rhythms drum-circle facilitator, chief-consciousness officer, light barrier, and forensic addiction certified therapist. Master drummer/percussionist with Agape International Spiritual Center. He was educated and trained by Jerry Bedlington and Angel Team Healings.

Hester, who is also a Vietnam veteran, volunteers with the Amity Foundation, a US-based organization dedicated to building community and preventing recidivism.